Pears, Grapes, and Dates
A Good Life After Mid-Life

Peter, May we all finish well (2 Timothy 4:7-8)

James Tonkowich

Copyright © 2015 James Tonkowich

All rights reserved.

ISBN-13: 978-1507872994
ISBN-10: 1507872992

DEDICATION

To Dottie

GROW old along with me!
The best is yet to be,
The last of life, for which the first was made:
Our times are in his hand
Who saith, ``A whole I planned,
Youth shows but half; trust God: see all, nor be afraid!"
    —Robert Browning

CONTENTS

Introduction	1
John	6
Pears	15
Grapes and Pruning	29
Grapes and Trellises	41
Dates and Their Roots	52
Dates and Sweetness	66
Epilogue	76

INTRODUCTION

And the wind shall say: "Here were decent godless people:
Their only monument the asphalt road
And a thousand lost golf balls."
　　　　—T. S. Eliot

Those three lines from T. S. Eliot's poem "Chorus from 'The Rock'" sum up my greatest fears about myself and my generation.

Having said that, you don't need to be in my generation to benefit from this book. We just happen to be the ones living life after mid-life today. Your turn will come sooner than you'd expect.

There are seventy-seven million (that's 77,000,000!) of us—the Baby-Boomers. And we've begun to retire in vast numbers. Since our births between 1946 and 1964, we've learned how to lead, to manage, to plan, to teach, to coach, to build, to write, and…. While we don't know how to do everything, as a group (again there are 77,000,000 of us) we can do just an enormous number of things and we can do them well. The wealth of experience, wisdom, and energy we Boomers represent is beyond calculating. It would, therefore, be an incalculable tragedy to squander that experience, wisdom, and energy in a "Golden Years" orgy of decent godlessness, road trips, and lost golf balls. Or at least I want to do more and get more than that out of whatever years I have left.

I suspect you do as well.

This book began as a series of journal entries from about ten years ago that somehow grew into an imagined dialogue between two fictional characters. I was a mere babe of fifty at the time pondering the next twenty or thirty years—or maybe a few more. Today it's more like the next ten or twenty years—or maybe a few more, but not many more. That "three score and ten" I've read about is getting closer by the day.

And while I'm a decent (though I hope not godless) person who is quite fond of road trips and has already lost at least a thousand golf balls, the American dream of retirement holds no appeal for me. Or at least the way it is so often lived holds no appeal for me. The reasons will become clear in the book, but the short version is: I've watched it and, far too often, it's a waste of time, talent, and treasure. And, yes, I can cite good examples of people I want to emulate. But still.

My wife's parents and my mother lived in over-50 communities in Florida. My mom worked into her eighties and (for the most part) loved it while my in-laws stopped working altogether. Their lives in those communities were good. They were comfortable, active, and happy. They enjoyed plenty of friends their own ages who were right there in the neighborhood. What they didn't have, however, were younger friends and as the friends their own ages began to die off one by one a deep loneliness grew with every funeral.

By contrast, my dad died before my mother moved to the seniors' development. He was seventy and he had his boots on. At the time, they lived in a neighborhood with all ages and went to church with all ages. Not surprisingly they had friends of all ages including my dad's students. He was one of the happiest, one of the best, and surely one of the best-loved community college adjunct faculty in history. His funeral service attested to it. It was packed with all ages including hundreds of his former and current students.

He died very much at peace—at peace with God, at peace with his family, at peace with the world, and (perhaps most difficult) at peace with himself. In those last professorial years of his life, he had a ball. He lived on the edge, teaching anything they threw his way whether had studied the subject before or not. Often he was only a chapter ahead of the students, but that was enough for him. It challenged not only his skills as a teacher, but his skills as a student too. He loved it and as near as I could tell, between teaching, my mom, and his grandson (our son), he was the happiest he had ever been.

On reflection, he lived out the ideas in this book though he died long before I began to write it. Which is another way of saying that I think I've captured some things that are tried and true. I just packaged them a bit differently as pears, grapes, and dates. How I arrived at images of fruit is impossible to say. I simply don't know, but it makes things easy to remember—and most of us need as much easy-to-remember as we can get.

As to proving them true in my own life, I'm still working on it convinced that what I've written really does point out the road to a good life after mid-life. It's actually rather simple, which, let the reader understand, is not the same thing as "easy." Swinging a golf club properly is simple, but if it was easy we wouldn't have all those lost golf balls, would we?

Pears, grapes, and dates teach lessons that are simple, but difficult, contrary to the way we've been trained to think and act, and contrary to the way our culture expects us to think and act. "Old age," as actress Bette Davis once said, "ain't no place for sissies." She wasn't politically correct perhaps, but you get the idea.

My wife, Dottie, and I have had numerous conversations between the two of us and with friends about "our next and maybe last great adventure." Dottie likes to quote George Bernard Shaw who said, "I want to be thoroughly used up when I die for the harder I work, the more I live." I prefer to quote gonzo journalist Hunter S. Thompson: "Life should not be a journey to the grave with the intention of arriving safely in a pretty and well preserved body, but rather to skid in broadside in a cloud of smoke, thoroughly used up, totally worn out, and loudly proclaiming 'Wow! What a Ride!'" Thompson and I have different ideas of what the "ride" should look like, but I appreciate the sentiment nonetheless.

I'm all for dying a dusty, tattered mess—with my boots on. How about you? How do we want to be used up? What's our next—even if it is our last—great adventure? How do we find peace while at the same time using all we've learned and experienced to make the world a better place for our children, grandchildren, and beyond? What can we do that stretches us beyond being decent, traveling the world, and losing another thousand golf balls?

Helen Keller, unable to see, hear, or speak, got it right: "Security is mostly a superstition. It does not exist in nature, nor do the children of men as a whole experience it. Avoiding danger is no safer in the long run than outright exposure. Life is either a daring adventure, or nothing."

That, in the final analysis, is what this book is about. I finished writing it years ago. The people who have read it enjoyed it and found it useful. I trust and pray you will as well.

JOHN

There is nothing which for my part I like better... than conversing with aged men; for I regard them as travelers who have gone a journey which I too may have to go, and of whom I ought to inquire whether the way is smooth and easy or rugged and difficult.
　　　　　　　—Socrates in Plato, *The Republic*

John always struck me as one of the sanest human beings I have ever met. He's intelligent, clever (not the same thing), and pleasant to be with. He's gentle, thoughtful, and incisive. And while "sane" is the word that spring to mind most readily, I suppose what I really mean is that seems to me that he's wise—not a word I'm very comfortable using. But John is wise—and old, not ancient, somewhere in his late seventies.

　　I, on the other hand, may or may not be old yet. And I'm quite certain I'm not wise yet—assuming that I'll ever be wise. I'm a middle-aged baby boomer from right about mid-boom and getting old had been on my mind at the time.

For one thing, I just celebrated another birthday. My comment about being able to feel the heat from the candles on my cake drew the predictable chuckle from the crowd of friends at my party (nearly all of them older than me), but in the back of my mind it bothered me. My birthday came along at a time when I was much too busy at work and immediately after a long weekend trip to Florida to visit my wife's parents at their retirement village. I mentioned to my father-in-law that I was turning fifty on Ash Wednesday. "Ah," he said, "then I guess you'll be giving up your youth for Lent." The whole month surrounding the birthday I was mildly depressed and so I decided it was time for a trip across the neighborhood to see John.

I first met John on a walk around the neighborhood twelve years ago. I was furious at something my wife, Sara, had said and I stomped out of the house in a rage taking the dog with me. Walking quickly, my head down, mumbling under my breath, and rapidly deciding to file for divorce, I crashed into John as he walked his dog. The collision knocked him down on the path and caused both dogs to bark and growl in anger.

He wasn't hurt badly by the fall—or rather, the landing—but it tore a hole his khakis. So after we got the dogs to calm down, I walked with him back to his house apologizing profusely. Once we got to his door, seeing the consternation on my face, John asked me what I was worried about. I blurted out that I wasn't worried about anything because I'd decided to get a divorce and all my problems would soon be solved. John began laughing, more, I think, from embarrassment than anything else. "Well," he said, "if that's so then life for you is much less complicated than mine has ever been. Why don't you come in and sit down for a moment. The dogs can rest and we can talk about that if you'd like."

I was so in need of someone to talk with that I jumped at this kind stranger's offer. So we sat down at his kitchen table with glasses of iced tea and muffins he had baked that morning. Two hours later I walked home to apologize to Sara and to begin cleaning up the mess.

Since then I've gotten used to going to see John when life seems overwhelming: at job changes, when my eldest went off to college, after my dad died. He listens carefully, asks questions, and adds things he's learned.

I hadn't been to see him for several months and I brought along a good bottle of red wine as a sort of friendship offering lest I seem like a foul-weather friend. I secretly wished he'd open it and we could sit down and share it over a long talk.

"Well," John said greeting me, "look at what the cat dragged in. Good to see you, Jeff. Good to see you. Come right in. For me?" he said taking the offered bottle. "Thank you. Thank you. Thank you."

The house smelled of latex paint and John's t-shirt and jeans were splattered with bright yellow spots. "I've been doing a little painting in my kitchen. Don't tell my daughter. She tried to take away my ladder years ago. I've just cleaned up so this a ideal time for you to stop by. Sit down and tell me how you've been."

"I've been okay," I said.

"'Okay'? Is that the best you can do?"

I filled him in on the details of the last weeks: work, birthday, and visit to my inlaws.

"What birthday is this for you?"

"Fifty."

"The big five-O upon you already."

"Like a lion on the neck of a zebra," I said dejectedly.

"Oh, dear," he answered, "that's a bit grisly. But why so sad? Fifty is a great decade. My fifties were probably my favorite time of my life. Although my sixties were lovely and my seventies are working out to be extremely pleasant." He paused. "Why are you so upset about getting old?"

"When I was in Florida, I met the Patio Guy."

"The Patio Guy?"

"When we were with Sara's parents, we stayed in an apartment in their retirement village. The patios of four of the apartments ran along the parking lot and I don't think there was more than four feet of grass separating those patios from the front bumpers of the parked cars. On one of the patios sat the Patio Guy." I sighed.

"He was sitting there when we left in the morning and when we returned in the afternoon." I continued, "He was there at noon one day when I had to run back to our apartment for something. All day long, there he sat on one of those $3.99 white plastic armchairs they sell at supermarkets. He was about two feet from the edge of the patio and equidistant from the sides. He sat and looked. He wasn't staring blankly out into space; he was just... looking."

"Well, maybe," said John, "he's recovering from a stroke. Stroke victims sometimes do that, you know."

"I guess that could be it, but I don't think so. We said, hello, one day and chatted briefly." I paused. "Who knows? Maybe he had just finished a tough assignment with the FBI, or put the final touches on his latest novel, or defended his dissertation finally fulfilling a life-long goal of earning a Ph.D. in particle physics."

"Oh, I like that last one best," John jumped in. "Or maybe he needed the kind of rest that you've told me that you enjoy on vacation smoking a cigar, sipping a beer, and sitting on a rock watching the tide come in along the Maine coast."

"Maybe."

"Or maybe he was just watching the world go by."

"If that's what he was doing," I said, "he picked the wrong place. Aside from three or four cars pulling into or out of the parking lot over the course of the day, the world doesn't go by his patio. And still he sat with nothing to see, nothing to do, not much to say."

I went on. "I know that the Patio Guy may be the most emotionally and spiritually healthy person I have ever met and I just don't realize it. Besides, we all need silence and solitude..." I trailed off.

"It's not that particular person that's got you upset," said John. "It's what you see in him. The Patio Guy—not the man himself—has become an image for you. Are you worried that you'll become the Patio Guy?"

"I don't want to get sedentary as I get older and I don't want to live like that ever. My boss…"

"Who's in his seventies and has jet fuel in his veins," added John.

"'…who's in his seventies and has jet fuel running through his veins' tells me about the men he sees moving to his upscale community also in Florida. These guys have been top executives for Global 2000 companies, senior partners at law firms, and successful physicians. After long careers in demanding jobs they've finally retired and moved to Florida. The future lies before them like some magnificent green valley full of possibilities. They've worked hard for years. Now they can let down and finally enjoy life. They can't wait to play golf or fish all day, every day."

"That sounds like a fine plan to most busy men I know."

"It always sounded like a good plan to me, but then he tells me the rest of their stories. Most of them play golf or fish every day for a while, but within eighteen months they're watching soap operas every afternoon. One of his neighbors and his wife can sometimes be seen grilling a steak for dinner at four in the afternoon."

"That's the ideal time," added John, "since the soaps are over and they'll finish dinner before the local news came on at five," he added facetiously.

"It gets worse. The two of them sit in lawn chairs near the gas grill, cocktails in hands watching the steak cook. *Watching the steak cook!* Could that be me someday?"

"It could be."

"But I don't want that to be me someday."

"And you're worried about it."

"Duh," I said in the sarcastic tone I'm used to hearing from my teenagers and then quickly apologized.

"No apology necessary. You're worried about a fruitless old age, about being like that bluegrass song:
'Old and in the way,' that's what I heard them say
They used to heed the words he said, but that was yesterday.
Gold will turn to gray, and youth will fade away
They'll never care about you 'cause you're old and in the way.
I used to worry about that too. All the time."

"But you're nothing like the Patio Guy."

"Well," he said, "I hope I'm nothing like the Patio Guy. Though I've had dinner at four in the afternoon on occasion and I've watched more than one steak sizzle on the grill."

There was a long pause.

"But, no," said John breaking the silence. "No, I'm not like that. I'm not like that on purpose. You see, I saw it coming too. I was an executive—you know that—and a pretty good one if I can blow my own horn. And when the time came, Maggie and I had already made a trip down to Florida to look at real estate for our retirement. We went to Arizona too for the same reason. We met wonderful people, saw old friends, and toured some lovely communities filled with beautiful homes.

"Now there's nothing wrong with retiring to Florida or Arizona. And there's nothing wrong with living in a retirement community. I have good friends in retirement communities around the country. But while it was all bright, shiny, and new, I could tell it wasn't for me. I saw Patio Guys too. And while I met plenty of active, happy, involved people, the Patio Guys scared me. 'Good heavens,' I thought, 'can't these people think of anything else to talk about other than their latest doctor's visit and what's on sale at the supermarket?' It wasn't the place for me."

"Exactly. What did you do?" I asked.

"Well, I continued to be the best executive I knew how to be and Maggie and I renovated and redecorated our house—this house. And I've lived here ever since even though after the kids left and Maggie died, there was no reason to have a place this big. When the time came to retire, I retired and stayed here to pursue life until it ends—and to be fruitful—to be involved in a positive way in the lives of others."

"You and Maggie renovated the place?" I asked.

"Yep."

I looked intently at him.

"You're thinking," he smiled, "that I renovated this house and in the process renovated my soul, aren't you?"

The thought had crossed my mind on many occasions especially since John continues his renovations with things like new paint. I hoped it wasn't true since I can barely hammer a nail and I have no intension of ever learning. The "home improvement projects" my wife is so fond of are torture for me.

"It wasn't the house." I was relieved. "No, it was the landscaping."

I tensed again. This was even worse.

He laughed. "I thought that would get a rise out of you. Not doing landscaping, but thinking about plants—the way they grow and ripen, age and bear fruit. You and I aren't the only living things on God's Earth that are aging. Snapdragons, spruce trees, and sweet corn age too." He laughed again looking a little shy. "You're not going to believe this, but I learned to get old by looking at plants."

"Plants?" I didn't believe him.

"Yep, plants. Not all plants. You see, I came across an old book my uncle had given me years ago. It was about horticulture, kind of an encyclopedia of plants and once I began reading it, I couldn't get enough. That sounds strange, but I learned long ago to give into those urges to know more about some odd subject. When that kind of urge comes over you and you want to study stars or birds or ancient history or plants, give in and do it because there's something in it. It's a sign of some sort, direction from above if you will. So, anyway, I read the whole thing and three plants stuck out as worth remembering. All these years later, I can't tell you much of what I read in that book, but I can tell you something about pears and grapes and dates. I've thought about them quite a bit."

I was beginning to suspect that my questions about getting older had come a bit too late. He had already slipped a cog. "Pears and grapes and dates?"

"That's right and, no, it's not dementia. You can calm down about getting older if you remember pears, grapes, and dates. You may even enjoy the process and you'll be fruitful."

"And what is it about pears, grapes, and dates that I should remember?"

"I'm glad you asked," he said. "I'm glad you asked. Let me open this lovely bottle of Pinot Noir and fetch two glasses. Then I'll begin."

PEARS

With full-span lives having become the norm, people may need to learn how to be aged as they once had to learn how to be adult.
—Robert Blythe

John returned with the open bottle, two glasses, and a plate of cut pears and Pecorino cheese. "I'll begin with pears," he said once he poured each of us a glass of wine, "because the lesson I learned from pears has to come first. Without this lesson, the others won't make much sense. Cheers," he said lifting his glass. He swirled the wine, breathed deeply, and took a sip. A big smile appeared on his face. "Ah, now that's good, very good. Thank you once again."

"My pleasure," I said also enjoying a sip.

"Now," he went on, "did you ever bite into a ripe peach only to be disappointed because it wasn't nearly as ripe as you thought?"

"Sure," I said, "You think it's ripe because it feels soft, but inside instead of being juicy and sweet, it's hard and crunchy inside. I hate that."

"Now, what about pears?" he asked picking up a slice, "Did you ever bite into a pear you thought was ripe only to find that it wasn't ripe at all yet?"

"No. The disappointment with a pear is that you think it's ripe and inside it's already turning brown."

"Exactly," he said smiling. "Peaches and most other fruit ripen from the outside in. Pears ripen from the inside out. As you get older, you've got to learn to ripen like a pear."

"Like a pear."

"Yes."

"From the inside out."

"Exactly."

"And how," I wondered aloud, "do I do that?"

"There's been dozens of books and probably hundreds of articles written about how shallow people are today," he began. "And in a culture like ours, one that's so centered on consuming, it's small wonder. We think life happens from the outside in and so if I want to change who I am, I go out and buy some new clothes or a new car. Do you have any idea how much is spent every year on cosmetic surgery? The new clothes, the new car, the new face, the new spouse—we somehow believe they'll make us new people."

"And, of course, advertising encourages that," I added. "A friend of mine needed a new car and found one that he liked, but it was, he said, 'skewed' too young for him. He's in his forties and the car is marketed as a car for people around thirty. He couldn't get himself to actually buy that model."

"So, what did he do?"

"He ended up with a luxury sports sedan skewed to successful guys in their forties."

"And there's nothing wrong with that as long as he hasn't convinced himself that a new car is going to change his life in some meaningful way. That's the mistake people make. All the moving and job changing people do. Why do they do it? Not all of it, but a lot of it happens, I think, because they believe they can change their lives from the outside. They think human beings are like peaches when, in fact, we're like pears—stupid pears, but pears nonetheless."

"How are we stupid?" I asked.

"We accept inadequate and dangerous definitions of ourselves. Advertisers and retailers call us 'consumers.' The computer people call us 'users.' It may seem like a small thing, but it affects the way we think about ourselves and others. You need to reject that nonsense about being a 'consumer' and a 'user.' It's nothing but an attempt to convince you that you can ripen from the outside in. Someone once said that we're human *beings*, not human *doings*. That's a little gimmicky, but I like it."

I thought for a second. I didn't quite know how to put what I wanted to say next. "But everybody already knows that."

"Really?"

"Sure. Or at least I know it. We need to concentrate on our inner lives, to do things like meditate, pray, and journal. Money can't buy happiness and we need to go within. In our materialistic culture, people are interested in spirituality."

"Good. I'm glad you understand. Now what are you doing to ripen from the inside out? How are you tending your inner life as you get older?"

"Well, I, er...." I was trapped by my own words.

"Nothing much really," I admitted. "Between the job, the house, my family, trying to get exercise, and paying the bills, I don't seem to find the time."

"And that," he said, "is why you don't have an answer. You will never—and I do mean *never*—'find' the time. You have to either *make* the time or there is no time. It's like the line from one of those *Star Wars* movies: 'Either do or don't do. There is no try.'"

"Well to tell you the truth, my kids have been driving me crazy lately—the older one who just started college especially. How am I supposed to develop an inner life with one teenager worrying me at college and another teenager in the house? Why should this mid-life kind of thing have to hit during their teen years. It hardly seems fair."

"Oh, it's more than fair. It's just as it should be. Listen," he said gently, "God has years and years to deal with your kids, but he's running out of time with you. You seem ripe enough on the outside. You're successful and you look it: a man in his prime showing confidence to your employer, your employees, your customers, and your friends. The problem is that, if you're like most people your age, you're not at all ripe inside and in spite of saying the right things, you haven't worked on your inner life at all.

"I've heard enough stories from you about raising your children," he continued, "to convince me that the solution isn't your kids growing up. The solution is for *you* to grow up. The fact that they're teenagers and hard to handle is just your wake-up call."

"What do you mean?" I was mildly offended, but I feared that he was right.

"Let's take one example. Your son dyed his hair blond last year."

"Yellow," I blurted out with annoyance. "He dyed his hair neon yellow. It practically glowed in the dark."

"Alright, alright, then, your son dyed his hair neon yellow. It glowed in the dark and you threw a fit. In fact, you're still angry."

"Why wouldn't I be angry?" I admitted. "The kid comes home with yellow hair, his grandparents are coming into town the next day for a big family wedding we're all attending that weekend, he's in the wedding party, and his yearbook photo was the next on top of it all."

"None of those things are worth getting angry about."

"Are you kidding?" I said with the anger boiling up in me all over again. "Explaining to my parents and all our relatives and friends about his hair? Having his picture with yellow hair in the wedding photos and yearbook forever? I was so embarrassed."

"Ah, so there it is."

"There what is?" I asked.

"The problem with the yellow hair was that *you* were so embarrassed?"

"Well, yes. I'm a leader in the community, my family was having a big event, and it just wasn't right for him to do that to me."

"Because, after all, it's all about you."

"What do you mean?" I said feeling the wind go out of my sails.

"I mean your son isn't in your equation. I mean that you acted—and you are acting—like the high school sophomore instead of the adult. Teenagers are hypersensitive about who they hang out with and what those people look like and how they look hanging out with those people. That's why teenagers don't like to go to the shopping mall with their parents. Right?"

"That seems to be the way the game is played," I replied.

"And that certainly is annoying, but it's okay for kids. No one expects them to be ripe. Their inner lives are, in large measure, unformed. But it's not fine for someone your age. What you've said is that you don't have the inner maturity to be seen with an immature son with neon yellow hair. After all, your parents and relatives won't approve. The hair is all so public. They might think you're a bad parent."

"They might," I said grudgingly. By now I knew he was right.

"And they'd be wrong. You're a good parent, but you still lack the inner maturity to get beyond the feelings of embarrassment we usually associate with high school. The outside of you is all dressed up like a ripe man, but deep down inside, you're still a teenager worried about how you look to others. Think back. Didn't you act like a kid in dealing with your kid?"

I thought back to an old girlfriend from tenth grade named Janet. We had a real thing going until Janet was in an automobile accident. Glass cut her in the face and she had a broken tooth. My extremely cute girlfriend looked terrible. And while I knew she'd heal up and be cute again, I broke it off. I didn't want to be seen with her and it still hurt when I thought about it. What a cruel, immature thing to have done.

As though he could read my thoughts, John said, "You've been doing that sort of thing for a long time, haven't you? People aren't quite right and you drop them."

"And partly I'm afraid," I heard myself saying, "that others will treat me like that…"

"…when you're 'old and in the way'?"

I nodded.

"Jeff, I get fearful about the same thing. We get older, slow down, slow down some more, and eventually we stop. And while we can and should prepare for that, it's frightening. Only a fool takes old age and death casually."

We were silent for a few minutes. "You know, Jeff," John continued, "you're too old to get away with being a peach. It's time to ripen like a pear."

"How do I do that?"

"You know, my son, Steve, is a writer," he said. "People find out what he does and want to know how they can become writers as well. 'What's the secret?' they ask him. 'There's no secret,' he tells them. 'If you want to be a writer, just start writing and don't stop.' 'But what should I write about?' they ask. 'Write about what you know,' he tells them, 'Just write about what you know.'

"I had no idea how to ripen from the inside out when I began. But I've never been one to let ignorance stop me. I made a commitment to grow my inner life and I just started with what I knew."

"What did you know?" I asked.

"Hmm," he said taking another sip of wine, "I have a better question. What do *you* know?"

"Not much except that getting old is bothering me."

"Good," he beamed. "You know enough to get started.

"Years ago," he went on, "when the kids were small, Maggie read a child psychology book. She got all excited about the developmental stages of children. She shared the stages with me ending with the teen years and one last stage: adult. I remember thinking that somehow more needed to be said. And, of course, it turns out that there's much more to be said. While I haven't studied the stages of adult development in any formal way, I've lived through most of them. The way I was thirty-two is about as similar to the way I am today as a seven year old is to a seventeen year old."

He paused, "You're worried about getting older because you've turned fifty."

"That's right," I said, "I really hadn't thought much about getting older until now."

"Turning fifty is one of the best things that will ever happen to you. At fifty, you're finally getting to where that inner life is so much less of a struggle. One friend of mine turned fifty and within weeks was writing poetry. He hadn't written a poem since some high school teacher assigned one. And his poems are good; they're thoughtful."

"He wrote poems because he turned fifty?" I asked.

"Not because he turned fifty. At fifty we cross some developmental line. We're finally ready to write poems. But it's not just poetry. I've kept a journal on and off since I was in my teens. It's funny to read what I wrote when I was… oh, how about twenty-seven. The entries are mostly factual: what I did, what I wanted to do, the data of my life. As I've re-read those journals, it's almost comical the things I thought were so important and took so seriously. That's one of the ways I know how much I've grown and changed."

"And your journal today?"

"…is about my life. Oh, I'm not saying that the facts aren't important. They are and I write down facts. But amassing facts leads you to believe that you can ripen from the outside in. 'If I do this or go here or have that, then my life will be better.' It might be more comfortable, but it probably won't be better. Of course, that wasn't even a consideration back then. I rarely asked, 'So what?' where today I ask it all the time."

"You never asked what the facts meant," I added.

"Correct, I hardly ever reflected on the facts. For example, I wrote about the birth of our daughter who nearly died in the delivery room. All the details were there and a few bits about how I felt and the beauty of life, but it was mostly facts. A couple of years ago, I began with those facts and wrote about Carrie's birth as if it had just happened all over again. I made connections that in my late twenties I never saw. There's so much to say about new life. And there's so much to say about long life—and death."

"So at age fifty we become more reflective."

"It happened to me and it happened to many others I've known. Of course lots of people run around entertaining themselves or watch TV and never notice, but my experience tells me that it's the case for nearly everyone. Are you getting more reflective?"

"It's hard to say," I began. "On the one hand, I haven't been writing poetry or journaling. On the other hand, things—normal, every-day things—seem to strike me as somehow different. Am I making sense?"

"Perfect sense. Go on."

"Last week when I got out of the car in the office parking lot I passed a stand of tulips—apricot colored tulips, big ones—in two beds near the front door to our office. The shape, the color, the brilliance stunned me. I crouched down to look at them more closely. I couldn't get over how beautiful they were with the sun shining on them. I didn't want to go into the building. I would have been content to stare at those flowers all day."

"What happened then?" he asked.

"One of my co-workers walked up and asked me if I'd lost anything. No, I said, I'm just admiring the flowers."

"And what did he say?"

"'Humm.'"

"Pardon?"

"'Humm.' He said 'Humm' and I felt kind of stupid."

"You felt stupid for admiring flowers?"

"It's not the sort of thing the company feels is a good use of executive time. Too inefficient. Shows you're not in control of your schedule."

"Ah," he said, "efficiency and control: two of the most highly overrated things in the world. Efficiency and control are the natural enemies of the inner life. They kill it off and must be avoided."

I laughed.

"I'm serious, Jeff. When I was still at my old company, I remember visiting a customer with a young salesman. The customer, Ray, was someone I had done business with for years and I was introducing him to the new guy. We had a great visit in his office and as we were leaving, my young colleague said to Ray, 'Call me any time you need me. I'm available 24/7.' That was a new turn of phrase then, one Ray had never heard. '24/7?' he asked. 'That's right,' said the new guy, 'You can call me twenty-four hours a day, seven days a week, holidays included.' There was a puzzled pause that just hung there a few seconds. 'Ray,' I said, 'don't even think about calling me 24/7.' 'Me either,' he said. And we both laughed. The new fellow forced a smile.

"When we got into the car to drive to our next appointment, he lit into me. I had embarrassed him in front of the customer and I showed the customer that I wasn't committed and that probably meant the company wasn't committed. 'You're the one with the stupid comment about 24/7.' 'Stupid?' he said, '24/7 is what it means to be in business today.' 'Really?' I said. 'I've been in business for years and no one ever expected 24/7 out of anyone. The only people I've ever heard of who are 24/7 are known as slaves.'"

"What did he say to that?" I asked laughing.

"He didn't really say anything. He mostly sat there with his mouth wide open and made funny little squeaky noises."

"I'm 24/7," I said soberly.

"Then you must be a slave," he replied.

"I must be, but it's the expectation. It's how we live."

"Look," he said calmly, "I don't have anything against working hard, but 24/7 will kill your inner life and probably ruin your health too. As we get older we need to be more and more in tuned to the rhythms of time and to our own limitations. Be available to people if you must, but leave it to the young and foolish to believe in 24/7. They're still caught up in the belief that they have control of their days and that efficiency and control are the be-all and end-all of life. Do you have any Jewish friends?"

"Excuse me?" The change of subject was a bit too abrupt.

"Jewish friends?" he repeated. "Do you have any?"

"Yes," I answered.

"When do they celebrate the Sabbath?" he asked.

"Friday night and Saturday."

"Exactly. Sundown on Friday until sundown Saturday is the Sabbath, the day of rest. You see, the Hebrew day begins with sunset. I think that's wise and wonderful beyond all telling."

"Why does it make a difference?" I asked puzzled.

"Simple," he replied. "In our typical way of thinking, the day begins when I get up in the morning. That puts a lot of pressure on me. I have to work hard all day because I'm responsible for the outcomes. I need to control my time and be efficient or else I'll loose out and it will be no one's fault but my own. If you're 24/7 it's even worse. Now you're responsible even when you're asleep because your day never begins or ends, it's just one giant now.

"The response to that is the Hebrew day. The day begins at sundown, when I go to sleep and I spend the first third of the day unconscious. I do nothing, accomplish nothing, and am aware of nothing. Instead I sleep and wake up in the middle of the day. And what do I find when I awake? I find that as I've slept, God has been at work. Because I don't start the day, I'm not responsible for it in the same driven way any more. I have to use my time well and get things done in an orderly way, but God has been at work and I wake to respond to God and join in on what he has already been doing. It's a wonderful way of looking at life."

"What does it have to do with the inner life?" I asked.

"If you have to run around being responsible for the day, you'll have no time for the inner life. You won't 'find' the time because you're too driven trying to take control and be efficient. Your focus will be outside and you'll try to ripen like a peach. In your rush, you'll think about your inner life and about God as add-ons—things you'll get to if you ever 'find' the time.

"But if God is the one who is ultimately responsible and your job is to respond by joining the work that began while you were unconscious, then not only do you have the freedom to *make* the time to develop your inner life, you have a need to make the time. It's a necessary investment in reality. Rather than control and efficiency, I can concentrate on what I need to do to be effective and than comes from inside

"So, am I in control? No, God is in control and I respond—a much better system than my being in charge all the time. And efficiency is something I no longer worry about. After all, I've slept through the first third of the day—so much for efficiency. I remembered that idea of day from Sunday school and from being with Jewish friends. My inner life took a huge leap forward when I discovered the wisdom in the Hebrew idea of a day. It allowed me to relax and grow."

We each drained our glass.

"So," I said still a bit unsure, "I still don't know what I need to do."

"There is no checklist of activities for growing an inner life, but if you must have a bottom line here it is: think about what you do and learn from it. That's what I try to do. I listen to my life. I read—not just newspapers, detective novels, and magazines—but some of the books that people for years have known can grow your soul: Augustine's *Confession*, *Pilgrim's Progress* by John Bunyan, and C.S. Lewis's children's books about Narnia—I read those to my children when they were little and I reread them every couple of years."

"I remember reading those to my kids too."

"And as I said earlier, I keep my journal. Try some of those things, especially the journal. Oh," he added, "and when something strikes me as good, I give thanks; when something I've done strikes me as bad, I ask forgiveness from God and others if I need to and then do what I can to make it right."

He paused.

"Do you think I should talk to my son about his yellow hair?" I asked looking at my hands. "You know, apologize for, well, the way I treated him. It was a couple of years ago, but somehow it's still here, still with us."

A bright smile rose on his face. "I suspect that it would make a big difference to him—and based on how you asked, I think it would make a big difference to you as well. You're getting older. It's time to take responsibility and to grow up. This is your opportunity to be a pear."

GRAPES AND PRUNING

Every man is the painter and the sculptor of his own life.
—St. John Chrysostom

The following Saturday afternoon I was back at John's door with another bottle of wine.

"All right," I said when he answered, "so much for the pears. Now tell me about grapes."

"My, my, I must have touched a nerve to send you back here so soon wanting more. Alright, let's talk about grapes, but to tell you about grapes," said John, "we're going to have to move to the back patio to enjoy this fine spring day and open this very lovely bottle of wine you were kind enough to bring over to encourage our conversation. Let's see 'Old Vines Zinfandel.' That should probably tell you something about grapes right there. No one ever boasts about 'new vines' Zinfandel."

We walked through the garage, out the back door, and under the arbor that led to John's back yard. The plants that surround the patio are full and lush in the summer. The flowers are bold and bright and more plentiful than mine have ever been. Now, however, in the spring, things seemed shrunk down. John had pruned his plants back—way back and the new growth was just beginning to hint at how the plants would fill out once again with green leaves and blossoms.

John slipped into the kitchen and returned with a corkscrew, two tall globular wine glasses as light as soap bubbles, a plate of Gouda cheese and water crackers and a plate bearing a bunch of grapes. He cut the foil on the bottle with a little knife, twisted the corkscrew into the cork, eased it out with a delightful "Pop," and poured a couple of ounces of the dark red zinfandel into each glass, offering one to me. I accepted it gladly.

"With thanks for life and all that sustains it," he said raising his glass.

"Amen," I answered not exactly knowing why.

We each took a sip and a thoughtful look came into John's face. "A bold cherry nose. Bright berry flavors with chocolate, pepper, and just the right amount of oak," he said. "Ah, grapes," he continued after a pause. "Who would ever think such wonderful and complex flavors could come from tiny Zinfandel grapes growing on old vines somewhere in Napa Valley. No one—I repeat—no one deserves wine this good. Thank you so much for sharing it with me. I am more spoiled now than ever."

"My pleasure," I said. "Tell me about the grapes."

"First tell me about your conversation with your son about his yellow hair."

I smiled. "When I brought it up, there was a combination of fear and anger in his eyes. Then when I apologized for how I had treated him, his eyes went soft, filled with tears, and he came over and hugged me. He hasn't done that in ages. I was so nervous about talking to him. I even put it off a day. When I finally just did it, it was great."

John smiled. "Good for you, Jeff—and good for your son to have you as a dad. That's the kind of ripening I was talking about."

He took a sip of wine. "That leads me directly into the whole matter of grapes. Grapes need to be pruned," he said. And then he looked at me, smiled, toasted me with his glass, and took another sip as if that's all he had to say.

"That's it?" I asked.

"That's it," he replied. "But that's a lot. You and I need to be like grape vines." He took another slow swallow of the wine. "One day my wife brought home a basket made from grape vines. They were very popular some years ago. I still have it. A great round thing. I couldn't believe that they were cutting down grape vines to make baskets, but, as it turned out, all someone did was find a profitable use for trash. It was recycling, that's all. Winemakers cut back their vines almost unmercifully. And that makes all the difference in the quality and quantity, the fruitfulness of the vine. We need pruning as well if we want to be fruitful."

"So how are we pruned?" I asked.

"Two ways. First, pruning comes our way whether we want it or not and, second, we need to learn how to prune ourselves. Proper pruning means that we, like grape vines, will bear more and better fruit the older we get."

"Pruning comes our way," I offered, "because we're getting older and can't do all the things we once could."

"Exactly," John answered. "There's an old book in the Bible that hardly anyone reads. It's a wisdom book called Ecclesiastes. People take a taste, don't understand it, think it's depressing, and stay away. That's too bad.

Through my fifties I fell in love with that book and it's become one of my best literary companions over the years. The book has a single clear—and intensely useful—message: Don't take yourself so seriously. We could all do with learning that.

"Anyway, at the end of Ecclesiastes there's a poem about getting old and the pruning that goes on. It talks about eyesight growing dim, hearing getting bad, teeth falling out, and memory fading; about being fearful all the time, napping all day, and waking up at the slightest noise in the middle of the night. And it goes on like that."

"And this is encouragement to you?" I asked.

"It's encouraging in part because it's so refreshingly honest. It's all going to happen, says the writer. In fact, it's all going to happen to *you* and so you better get used to the idea and 'Remember your Creator in the days of your youth.' He keeps coming back to that thought: remember your Creator. Develop an inner life to go along with the pruning of age and accept that pruning when it comes. I've got glasses, a hearing aid, and a couple of pieces of plastic in my gut where they repaired a hernia. I nod off from time to time during the day and in the middle of the night I wake up. I'm a much lighter sleeper than I used to be. While I still have all my teeth, spicy food and I parted ways long ago. My memory is still sound, but I wonder how long that will last. I've also got a few more wrinkles than I had when I was thirty. I was better looking then if I'm any judge. Besides, I could run for miles. I even finished a marathon. I loved that until my knees got so bad that I had to give it up. And, of course, Maggie died and a big part of me fell by the wayside. Life prunes you and you have no choice but to accept it."

"Shouldn't we fight all that?" I asked.

"Fight? I'm not sure that's the right word because I don't know what it means. Maggie died. There was nothing to fight. My knees got bad. Who do I argue with? Certainly we should do our best to keep ourselves in good shape and take care of our bodies, minds, and spirits as best we can, but how can you 'fight' getting older? Oh, people try things like face lifts, tummy tucks, botox, and other things that allow them to pretend they're not getting older, but let's face the facts: the years pass and no amount of fighting makes them stop."

"You mean that old age—and I guess even death—are part of life so we should just go with the flow."

"Aging is certainly part of life and I guess death is too. It's the final snip of the pruner's sheers. It's when earthly life itself is pruned from us. Neither of us is there just yet, but the way to prepare is to understand that you're getting older, 'Remember your Creator in the days of your youth,' and prune. Those who want to pretend it isn't happening are kidding themselves and are in for a rude awakening."

He took a thoughtful sip. "What I mean when I talk about being like a grape vine is that you need to take care of yourself by taking the pruning of age into consideration. My knees went out and I couldn't run. So I began to walk for exercise. My eyes got bad and I got glasses. My hearing has gotten weak and so I got a hearing aid. My metabolism slowed down suddenly six or seven times during my life beginning when I was about twenty. I ate like… well, like a fifteen year old when I was fifteen. When I turned twenty, I kept eating like that and, much to my surprise, I put on weight. So instead of going on eating like I was fifteen, I ate less. When it happened again, I changed my diet again and again. People get fat and flabby as they age and I think it's an indication that they're not responding well to life's pruning. And I don't say that because of the physical problems associated with weight, but because they don't seem to understanding how life works. Life pruned them and they're going along as if nothing new has happened."

"Because they're not pears?" I offered.

"Not always, but in many cases, yes. They're not ripening from the inside. If your inner life isn't ripe, you won't have the wisdom required to know what to do when you're pruned."

"My spare tire is the result of the last metabolism change I never quite adjusted to. It's not very pleasant to make the necessary changes."

"Well, pruning hurts," he answered. "Having part of you cut off is never pleasant, but it's the way to fruitfulness, the way to avoid being 'old and in the way.'"

"So most of the pruning relates to health?" I asked.

"No, not at all. When your children finally grow up and move out of the house, you've been pruned and, oh, my, how it hurts. The years shape the relationship we have with our children and we can't do much about it. Once they grow up, we have no choice but to accept them back as friends with whom we have a long history. The only alternative is to try to hang on to them as children with the predictable result that we make a mess of everyone's life."

"Your kids live far away, don't they?"

"One across the country, one in Europe, and one nearby. Those European grandkids are so far away—it hurts even to think about them; I miss them so much. So I have a choice: I can either be bitter and angry about it or I can see them and enjoy them as much as I can. I write to the kids and grandkids every week. Not e-mail, but plain old fountain pen and paper."

He paused to take another sip of wine. "Ah, grapes," he sighed. We sat silent for a moment longer.

Then John spoke again, "Grapes can only *be* pruned; they can never prune themselves. We can and that's an important point to make."

"Isn't that what you've been talking about?" I asked. "We get old and prune ourselves accordingly."

"No," he replied, "That's not it. Up till now, I've been talking about graciously responding to the pruning that life hands us. This is something different. As we age we have to cut back our own excessive growth."

"Like what?" I asked with some hesitancy.

"I'll begin with what I think is the big one: bitterness. The reason we hear so much about bitter old people is that a lot of old people are bitter. That's the primary reason I do my best to spend time with young people although it's pretty easy to pick out the ones who will be the bitter old people of the future. Sad really.

"Before my father died, he lived here with Maggie and me. Dad throughout his life was a very meek, mild, quiet man. He never made a fuss, never raised his voice, never seemed to get angry. And then he got old and sickly."

"What happened then?" I asked.

"Well, his memory for most things began to fade and as that happened his whole personality seemed to change. He went from meek and mild to bitter and angry. Bit by bit old memories surfaced, memories of every slight, every insult, every unpaid debt. And his feelings about the people in his past—and some in his present—came into his mind and ran right out of his mouth in wave after wave of verbal venom. Under the meek, mild, old-duffer exterior there were long, thick bitter branches bearing what I began to think of as poisonous fruit. When he got so sick that we couldn't care for him, we put him into a nursing home. There even more came out. Family and friends who went to see him were shocked and after a while nobody went to see him because no one wanted to hear the bitter, angry, unforgiving words. And there he was: not only bitter, but alone. And that's the way he died." He took another sip. "To this day, that scares me half to death. 'Like father, like son'? Dear God, I hope not."

"But," I protested, "you're not like that."

"Ah, but I am—or at least was and, who knows, I may still be. By which I mean, I sincerely hope I've pruned away most of the old festering bitterness, but I really don't know that I have. It takes hard, constant, and concentrated attention. At least," he reflected, "I think I've gotten rid of some of it."

"What do you mean, 'gotten rid of some of it'?"

"I mean that I got out my pruners and began looking for all the bitterness I could find. I went on an internal seek-and-destroy mission. In your youth you can get away with being a little bitter. It's poison, but it won't kill you—at least not right away. The older you get though the more you need to find the bitter shoots and prune them before they poison your life and the lives of those around you."

For reasons I can't explain, my mind raced back to college and the underhanded way a guy named Todd stole my date for a formal dance. Linda was going with me. I had asked her a month earlier and she said, yes. Then, a week before the big day, she announced that she was going with Todd who had weaseled his way between us. I could feel my pulse increasing and my blood pressure increase the second I pictured him. My stomach began to knot up as well. I could just....

John was looking right at me. "You don't want to get old with that sort of thing still in your mind and heart."

"But how do I get rid of it?"

"All I can tell you is how I did—or rather what I'm doing—and that may help."

John refilled our glasses. We both sipped. "Old vines Zinfandel. It only got this good because it was pruned."

We munched some Gouda and crackers.

Finally he spoke. "I got a notebook, a pen, and a mentor—a spiritual advisor, if you like. I found someone who was, if not wise, at least discreet. Someone to whom I could tell my angry secrets."

"Someone older than you?" I asked.

"Actually it was someone quite a bit younger, my pastor from church. I told him what was on my mind and he suggested the notebook and pen. As I told you last week, I've been keeping a journal for years, but this was something new for me. I'd sit down each morning, think about my life from one age to the next, and look for bitter shoots. They were all over the place when I started: the elementary school playground, the high school basketball team, college classrooms, board rooms, golf courses, tennis courts, Maggie and my bedroom, and highways all over the country. I'd been wronged and no one apologized and, to my shock, I was still furious. After more than sixty years, I was still angry over being called out when I was safe on the winning run in a kick ball game. It wasn't fair. I was the worst kickball player who ever darkened the third grade and my moment of vindication and glory was stolen from me. Can you believe it?"

I thought again about Todd. "I can believe it. So what happened when you dredged up all that stuff?"

"I wrote it down in my notebook. I began writing

narratives about what happened, but then I switched to writing dialogues."

"Between the offender and yourself?"

"No," he said. "Between myself and myself. I'd write out the hurt and then write out the counsel to let go, to remember how much I've been forgiven and forgive. It was a bit like talking to my own grandchild. The young me would complain and rant and then the grandfatherly me would try to put it into perspective. I wrote pages and pages, story after story. I was like my dad spewing venom, but in a controlled way in private, not out in public. And I had a specific goal: I was cutting off bitter shoots. Then once every two weeks I'd go visit my spiritual advisor and tell him what I learned."

"What did he do?"

"He listened and reminded me of what theologians call grace: because God sacrificed to forgive me, I can sacrifice to forgive others. I could give up my right to be angry, my bitterness."

"It sounds like we're back to ripening from the inside out."

"We are. Pruning is part of growing up and ripening."

"I've tried to forgive people from my past from time to time, but it's so hard."

"Oh, it's a struggle to this day for me. 'Forgive others from your heart' is very simple and very difficult. That's why you need a mentor, someone who can talk you over the hurdles and help you remember what St. Augustine said 1,600 years ago."

"What was that?" I asked.

"Augustine taught that evil deeds—sins—are their own punishment. That helped me to do a lot of forgiving."

"I don't understand," I said shaking my head.

"When I'm stuck unable to forgive, I remember that the person who stole from me or lied to me or cheated me is someone who deserves my compassion. One of the penalties for bad behavior is behaving badly. You see, he did more damage to himself by his actions than he ever did to me. When we treat people badly, cheat, or steal, we damage ourselves."

"How's that?"

"When we sin, to use Augustine's language, we ruin our character and actually become a little less human. When we forgive, we act with God's magnanimity and so become more human."

I thought about Todd again. After college he and Linda got married. He went to an Ivy League business school, got a great job, rose up the corporate ladder, and then went to prison for embezzlement. Linda divorced him. As I thought about him in those terms, my anger seemed to subside—at least for the moment.

John was looking at—or possibly through—me over his glass of wine. "Prune away that anger that's grown into bitterness and throw it out. Then you can work on your fear."

"Fear? This is starting to sound like a twelve-step program."

"Maybe it is. Do you think addicts are the only people who are controlled by anger and fear? Those two run our lives more than most of us can imagine and we need to prune them back before they take over."

He drained his glass. "Aah! Wonderful things, grapes. And now, I'm being pruned."

"What?" I laughed.

"I can no longer drink wine in the afternoon and not be expected to take a nap. That was one of the best bottles I've had in years and I fully expect the result will be one of the best naps I've had in years."

"But what about the dates?" I insisted.

"Calm down," said John. There'll be plenty of time for dates some other day. And I've got more to say about grapes first and I want to take my time. I'm too tired just now. Besides, you've got plenty to think about with pears and grapes. Have you begun journaling?"

"No," I said, " and I'm going out of town this next week."

"A road trip! What an excellent time to begin," smiled John. "Go buy a notebook and pen to take with you. Unplug the hotel TV, write about pears and grapes, and do some pruning. Then come back soon and we'll talk again. You can tell me what you've learned and I'll prattle on some more about grapes."

"Agreed," I said.

GRAPES AND TRELLISES

I once asked an old priest, a famous spiritual director, what he had learned from hearing thousands of confessions. He had a ready answer: "There are no grown-ups." There are grown-ups who pretend, and then there are those who have grown up to know the "second naïveté" of our utter dependence.
—Richard John Neuhaus

"John," I said when he answered the door, "this journaling has me more upset than ever."

"Why? What have you written?" he replied as he ushered me in. He had a look of real concern on his face.

"That's the problem," I answered. "I haven't written a blessed – or cursed – thing. But I've doodled quite a bit."

Then he began to laugh. "When you phoned," he said, "I thought there was a real problem." He laughed again. "Jeff, if the worst you can tell me is that you were doodling instead of writing, I'm afraid I can't be too concerned. I thought you'd made some terrible discovery about your life."

"I did," I said, "I discovered that even though I'm turning fifty, I'm no poet. This isn't working for me."

"Oh, I doubt either of those statements are true. I think you just don't know where to begin. The fact that you keep coming to my door is at least some indication that it's 'working'—whatever that means. Here, come with me."

He led me into his den and motioned me to a worn leather armchair. "You sit there and calm down and I'll be right back," he said as he headed toward the kitchen.

I looked around. The room was lined with bookcases nearly filled up with books. I remembered how my mother used to arrange books by how tall they were. John's books were arranged by topic and by author. Sets, instead of being together on one shelf were spread around based on the content of each volume. The coffee table and the floor near my chair were stacked with books as well. On top of the coffee table pile was a notebook and fountain pen.

When John returned he had two small wine glasses, a cold bottle of Pinot Grigio, some Swiss cheese, and an apple he had cored and cut into pieces. He sat down and I immediately apologized. "I'm so sorry. I had every intention of bringing you another bottle of wine. Please forgive me."

"Forgive you?" he responded. "Why should you apologize and why should I forgive you when all you've done is to give me the opportunity to be hospitable to a favorite guest?"

"I just don't want to be a bother, that's all."

"Why would you think you're a bother?"

"Well, I take up your time and have questions and needs and… well, I don't want to be a burden or anything."

"And somehow if you bring me gifts, then you're not a burden?"

"Well...," I began to feel my face redden. "I suppose I'm a little less of a burden. I feel like I'm giving back."

"You're still struggling with the very same thing you and I first talked about. You never want to be a burden and so you believe that you have to trade. That *does* make the prospect of old age frightening. Sooner or later you have nothing to trade – or so you imagine – and then the sky falls because you become 'old and in the way' – a burden. That may also be the reason words don't come when you journal. You're stuck on that one thought."

He poured the wine and handed me a glass. I took it, but continued to stare at my knees.

"Here's to being a burden to others," he said as he raised his glass. "It's what living in this world is all about."

I lifted my head and stared. John was smiling with a twinkle in his eyes.

"Oh, I'm very serious," he said as if reading my mind. "Either you're a burden to others or you're long dead. Even the newly dead are a burden, you know. To be alive is to be a burden to others. That's the second truth about grapes. Grape vines are a burden. It's the only way they can grow and produce fruit."

"What do you mean?" I asked.

"I mean that before a vintner plants his grape vines he needs to prepare his vineyard. So he cultivates the soil and installs a system of trellises. Every vineyard has them, usually fence posts all in rows strung with stout wires between them to support the vines. After the harvest in the fall, the vines are pruned back to their trunks. Then when spring arrives the vintner looks for the new shoots and ties them to the wires so that as they grow, the branches and later the grapes are suspended by the trellis. Or to put in another way, the vine and its fruit are a burden to the trellis. You can't grow good grapes without that simple fact."

"That's fine for grapes, but aren't we humans supposed to take care of ourselves? As we grow aren't we supposed to become self-sufficient? That's what being an adult is all about. You grow out of childhood and instead of being cared for, you care for others—they become your burden. Then you get old and suddenly you're a burden again."

John sighed. "Most people believe that," he began, "I think it's a gigantic lie. It's the 'myth'—if you'd prefer that word to 'lie'—of self-sufficiency. In the final analysis it's all smoke and mirrors. There's no such thing as self-sufficiency and people would be a whole lot happier if they understood that.

"Let me tell you about a fellow I knew years ago," he continued. "His name was Dan and he had been a genuine actual flower child."

"You mean a hippie?" I asked.

"No, not a hippie. He always insisted that he wasn't one of those. According to him hippies came along later. He was a flower child.

"Dan was born down south somewhere—Tennessee, I think. I don't believe his family farmed for a living, but they lived well off the beaten path on a mountain and did work the land some. They also spent quite a bit of time hunting and fishing. Anyway, Dan grew up with lots of animals. He learned how to milk cows and goats and how to handle horses, burros, and mules as farm animals."

"Do you mean plowing with them and all?"

"That's exactly what I mean. What farming his family did, they did without tractors or other modern machinery.

They only used animals. And Dan loved it. He loved it because, as far as he was concerned, animal powered farming was the way to become self-sufficient. And self-sufficiency was Dan's overriding goal in life at the time. I don't remember if he told me why, but he did say that what he longed for more than anything else was to have enough land to work and enough success in working that he didn't need anyone else in the world."

"But wouldn't he need other people for say new plows or new axe heads or knives or rope or a thousand other things?"

"The ability to trade was a part of his vision of self-sufficiency. But I agree with what you're probably thinking: his goal was unattainable because human life isn't that way. But he didn't believe it at the time and his sights were set on self-sufficiency.

"Anyway, he pursued his goal to San Francisco and…"

"To San Francisco?" I interrupted. "Was he going to start farming in the middle of Union Square?"

"No. He went to San Francisco, specifically to the Haight-Ashbury district, because he heard about the gathering of the flower children. According to him the flower children were all about getting back to nature and being self-sufficient. You know: sharing a commune, living off the land, and enjoying peace and love together forever. 'Getting back to the Garden' they called it using biblical imagery.

"So off he went to San Francisco and arrived in the spring of 1967 in time for the 'Summer of Love.' I remember reading about the hoards of young people, the music, the free love as they called it, and, of course, the drugs. What I didn't know was the part Dan told me. The Summer of Love was the prelude to a great agrarian dream. At the end of the summer there was a big parade in San Francisco to celebrate the dawning of a new age. The flower children were the first wave of a new humanity and they marched out of San Francisco into communes out in farm country. The hippies—a pale reflection of the true flower children according to Dan—moved into Haight-Ashbury after the main event. The flower children were out in the country by then 'getting back to the Garden' as fast as they could.

"Well, as you can imagine, Dan's knowledge and skills were invaluable to this project. He knew how to farm without power equipment and he could do it all organically to top it off. But as you probably know, farming, even if you have all the latest tractors, milkers, and other tools, is hard work."

"Oh, I know all about it," I said, "As a teenager I spent a summer on my uncle's dairy farm up in Wisconsin. I've never worked so hard in my life. Up with the sun, out milking, then cleaning up the mess the cows made as they were milked—and all that before breakfast. Then the chores went on till sundown and mucking out the barn fafter the evening milking. And it's like that seven days a week all year long."

"I can tell from that expression on your face," laughed John, "that you're grateful for other career options that surfaced."

"It was the kind of job every kid should have at least once during high school or college to put things into perspective. While I appreciate what my uncle and all his fellow farmers do for us, that life was not the life for me."

"Well," John continued, "as it turned out that life wasn't the life for the flower children either. Most of the people on the commune with Dan were suburban or urban kids. About the closest any of them got to farming was cutting the lawn. This was real farming: clearing land, plowing, cultivating, planting, tending, fertilizing, and on and on. And remember they did it all with animal power so you have to include taking care of the animals and all their gear. It wasn't like feeding the dog; it was a huge undertaking.

"Dan told me that he worked all day every day from sunup to sundown. Meanwhile, his fellow farmers pitched in when they had a mind to. Mostly they hung out playing music, getting stoned, and enjoying the 'free love.'"

"So what you're saying is that given the choice between back-breaking physical labor for twelve hours a day on the one hand and drugs and sex and rock 'n' roll on the other, most people chose drugs and sex and rock 'n' roll. Now there's a shocker."

"That sums up Dan's story of the commune rather nicely. You've always had a way of simplifying complex issues, Jeff." He tipped his glass toward me in a toast and we both took a sip of the crisp, citrusy wine.

"As you might imagine," John went on, "Dan became increasingly frustrated and finally left the commune after he realized that nothing was likely to change. The self-sufficiency he had in mind would have to be found elsewhere." He paused. "I'm trying to remember where Dan went from the commune. Hmm. Well, it really doesn't matter. Eventually he ended up in Colorado living in a cabin up in the Sangre de Christo Mountains—the Blood of Christ Mountains—tending goats."

"Goats?" I asked.

"Yes, goats. Strange to think about here in our little neighborhood, but someone has to take care of the goats or we'd have not goat cheese and that would be a pity. If I had some, I'd serve it. It would go well with this wine, don't you think?

"Anyway, Dan loved goats. They were, in fact,

something of a symbol of his quest for self-sufficiency. 'John,' he once told me, 'if you leave a herd of a hundred goats out in the Rockies over the winter, come spring you'll still have eighty or more. Leave a flock of a hundred sheep out and they'll all be dead long before Christmas.'

"The sheep need a shepherd to care for them; they're a burden. The goats will care for themselves; they're self-sufficient. And so Dan identified with goats and happily tended them in the southern marches of the Rocky Mountains. He had a big garden, did some hunting, preserved vegetables and meat for the winter, chopped wood, and did a little trading in the nearby town for whatever he needed that he couldn't produce for himself. His dream, he told me, had finally come true. He was self-sufficient. He was no longer a burden to anyone."

John fell silent as we both sipped our wine and nibbled on cheese and fruit. "And then the other shoe dropped?" I asked.

John smiled. "It sure did. Dan had come down his mountain just before the snows to do a little last minute trading in town. He needed kerosene for his lanterns and a few other supplies. He went from store to store and was on his way back to the road home when someone shot him in the leg."

"Some one shot him?" I asked startled. "Why?"

"Apparently there was no reason. It was someone who was known as being kind of crazy and who was drunk at the time. He had a gun, Dan was walking by, and I guess shooting him seemed like a good idea at the time. Anyway, the bullet made a clean path through Dan's thigh. They treated him and he spent a night or two away from his cabin—and his dream. He couldn't wait to get back and so someone drove him home in the back of a pickup and left him there."

"You know," I interrupted, "you make this story sound like he had no friends."

"He didn't. That's one of the ugly little facts about self-sufficiency: it creates isolation and loneliness. 'I don't need you' or 'I *won't* need you,' isn't a particularly good basis for a relationship."

I've thought about that more than almost anything else John said to me.

"Dan had nobody and the winter was just beginning. Up in his cabin his dreams of self-sufficiency were rapidly falling apart. The days were short and there were lots of chores to do in daylight. The problem, of course, was his leg. Even years later when I knew him he walked with a limp and he said that at the time pain was with him everywhere he went. Getting his supply of water was a daily torture of walking and hauling. The animals needed care. Wood still needed chopping. And the nights were long.

"His only comfort, he said, was a transistor radio. And because he really was lonely and wanted human conversation, he listened to a station that played Bible teachers. To conserve the batteries, he limited himself to a half hour a day when he listened to one particular old-time preacher who sooner or later got around to talking about sheep and goats. The preacher said that God's preference is for the sheep. And so in the spring Dan left his cabin to rejoin the human race and be a burden to others."

"But," I protested, "isn't it important to be independent of others even if we're not self-sufficient?"

"No," John answered. "If anything I think it's dangerous and unhealthy. Independence is an aggressive stance toward others. It sees everyone as the other and will only interact with those others on its own terms."

"Come on," I said, "it's not that bad. It's just that you want to have something to offer to the relationship."

"Even worse," he countered. "Now all relationships are contractual, a matter of bartering, of swapping goods and services. You bring the wine; I'll let you in and talk with you. It turns other people into commodities and every relationship into a commercial endeavor. That way, when you're old or terminally ill, unable to bring something to the table any more, you end up excluded from the game altogether. And so we victimize the very people who we should be looking after, the weak and the infirmed. They end up feeling 'old and in the way' because in this system that's exactly what they are.

"The grape vine depends on the trellis and in that relationship of interdependence, the grape vine does what it was created for: producing good grapes, and the trellis does what it was created for: supporting grape vines. I'm not your friend because of a couple of bottles of good wine or because of your time that I know is precious or because of some status your visits bestow on me. And I hope I'm not your friend because I give you the time you need to think about your life and dispense what may or may not be helpful ideas."

"Not at all," I said quickly. "I enjoy being with you and I appreciate your friendship and hospitality."

"But you still feel badly for not bringing something to trade."

I began to protest, but John put up his hand to silence me. "Jeff, when you look to me for help, your humanity is responding to my humanity. When I answer, it's the same thing: my humanity responding to yours. And humanity is not something that appears one day and goes away on another. It's something you have from the very beginning to the very end. That's why your mother took care of you from the moment she realized she was pregnant. That's why your parents cherished you and looked after you at each stage of childhood. That's why Sara loves you and your kids love you. And that's why you deserve to be cared for and loved into your old age and to your dying day. And it's why even your corpse should be treated with reverence and respect. Not because you can trade, but because you're one of us: a human."

"And all those old folks who die alone?"

"They're some of the saddest people of all because their humanity has been violated by others. And the ones who won't take care of them are sadder still since they violate their own humanity by their indifference. They believe the lie of self-sufficiency and it cuts them off from others—except, of course, when they can trade. Sooner or later self-sufficiency will betray them just as it betrayed my friend Dan. He was fortunate that it betrayed him early in life. When he found out about the lie, he began bearing the burdens of others, letting himself be a burden to them. Most people seem to learn when it's too late if they learn at all. I told you about caring for my dad as he got old and what a burden—and a pest—he was."

"Yes, that's quite a story."

"Well, hard as it was to put up with his anger and negativity, it was okay. It's what you do for other humans. Sometimes you're the vine and sometimes you're the trellis."

He fell silent and I looked at the age in his face. "Thanks, John," I said.

He smiled. "Now why don't you try journaling again? Start by making a list of the people who have supported you and the people you've supported and give thanks for them all."

DATES AND THEIR ROOTS

A man travels the world over in search of what he needs and returns home to find it.
—George Moore

Over the next few weeks, I finally did what John had suggested: when I was out of town, I wrote. For a couple of days I fretted about what kind of notebook and pen I needed, but finally bought a simple spiral bound notebook and a roller ball, sat down, and began to write—usually in the evening at a hotel room desk.

The hardest part was getting started—actually sitting down to write. I knew it was a good idea, but it seemed that anything and everything had power to keep me from my task. Keeping the televisions in the hotels turned off was probably the biggest challenge. I never watch much television at home, but walking into a hotel room and surfing the cable channels had become a habit. Nonetheless, if I could keep the tube off and actually get started, the words began to come rather easily.

I thought and wrote about my marriage, my job, my friends, and all sorts of other people and issues in my life, but most of all I thought and wrote about my kids. John was right. Too often I found myself embarrassed by them and that's why I got angry. It was time to grow up rather than resenting "how they made me look." It was time to drop my other resentments as well—schoolmates, fraternity brothers, old girlfriends, business associates, and customers all came to mind. There were too many faces that part of me wanted to smack while part of me just wanted to forgive. I also cut down on snacks and deserts and went for longer more frequent walks. I had put on a dozen or so pounds and now was the time to prune away that extra baggage as well.

It was about a month later that I showed up at John's house with another bottle of old vines Zinfandel and my notebooks.

"Welcome, welcome. And a bottle of Zin! Ah, and from noble, fruitful, *old* vines!" he said. "And notebooks? More than one?"

"Well, I kind of got going and, to be honest, my handwriting is kind of huge," I said as he flipped through a notebook.

"Oh, my, yes. You know at your age, reading glasses are a good idea."

"They're right here," I replied pulling half-frames out of my jacket pocket. "I have them, but my wife refers to them as my 'old guy glasses' so I'm really not that interested in wearing them."

"'Vanity, vanity, all is vanity,'" he said, "Let's be honest, my friend, that's exactly what they are: old guy glasses for...well, for old guys."

"Thanks so much," I said.

"Not at all," he replied, "Think nothing of it. Anyway I've been looking forward to your visit for a couple of days now and I bought us something to eat. How well it will go with the wine, I don't know, but it's the appropriate thing to serve."

He motioned me to his old leather wing-backed armchair, the back darkened by decades of heads leaning against it, and I sat down among the books while he went off to the kitchen. Soon he returned with glasses, a corkscrew, and a plate piled with cheese, crackers, and dates. He cut the foil, uncorked the bottle, and poured the wine.

"Ah," he said swirling the deep red liquid around the glass and holding it to the light. He breathed the aroma deeply and took a sip. "Old vines again. Nobody but nobody deserves wine this good. I am surely one of God's most spoiled children. But then, I've said that before, haven't I?"

"You have," I laughed.

"Well," he said after a moment, "it bears repeating on a daily basis since we're all so quick to forget and think we deserve. It's all a gift, you know."

He reached to the plate on the table in front of us and picked up a date. "The date," he proclaimed as he held it aloft. "The humble, homely date." He stared at it for a moment. "You've been kind enough to sit through a fruity old man's dissertation about pears and grapes and now we'll press on."

"I thought that was a 'fruit*ful* old man.'"

"Oh," he said, "fruit*ful* I pray and fruity I know. Regardless, you've returned to hear about dates."

"That's the third fruit?" I asked.

"That's the third fruit," he answered. "Not much to look at," he said examining it again, "and not many people outside Thousand Palms, California, pay much attention to it, but the date says a great deal about getting old. You see the tree this little brown beauty grew on was probably very old. Date trees live a long time and I learned two things from those trees." He paused popping the date into his mouth.

"And they are...?" I urged.

"Number one: grow roots—long, deep, vital roots. Dates live in the desert, in brutal conditions especially for a great, tall tree. The desert is dry and harsh. And it's not a big secret that in order to live there, they need to be rooted."

"To get water?"

"Yes, to get water, but also to keep from being blown over. The winds out in the desert are fierce. They can push date palms nearly horizontal. Without deep, strong roots, the trees would rip out of the ground. See that flower bed?" he asked pointing out the window.

"The one with the yellow snapdragons?" I replied.

"That's it. That flowerbed used to be an oak tree. About seven years ago, we had that wet summer and then a hurricane. Do you remember that year?"

"Sure," I said. "Trees were down all over the area. You lost a big oak in that storm?"

"I sure did and it missed the house by a hair. I watched it fall from this window. When I went out to look at the damage, I was shocked. I thought oaks were well rooted, but those roots weren't nearly as deep as I imagined. When the rains came and the wind blew, the roots ripped out of the ground and over went the tree. Date palms don't do that."

"Well, there's no rain where they live."

"That's true, but nonetheless, the winds blast the trees and their deep roots allow them to spring back once the storm passes by. You and I need to be anchored like that. We need roots if we're going to stand up to the winds. 'Winds of time'—sounds a bit melodramatic and more than a bit cliché, doesn't it? But that's exactly what blows at us and we need roots as we age."

"That's kind of counter-cultural, isn't it?" I asked. "I mean, isn't the story of our modern rootlessness legend by now."

"Oh, absolutely," he replied. "Modern people are rootless, but if you and I are going to grow old in such a way that we don't become cranky and unhappy old curmudgeons or lonely wanderers, we're going to have to buck the trend and put down roots. And there are at least four areas of root growth that need to happen. The first is your marriage."

"My marriage?" I said.

"I'm amazed," he began, "with the number of 'suddenly single' folks there are at older and older ages. Widowhood happens, but people in their fifties and sixties are divorcing. I think it's crazy. Well, more sad than crazy, I guess. The older you get, the more you need old friends. I can't see the sense in cutting off the one person who is probably your oldest friend, the person who knows you best."

"Maybe if you don't want to be known that well it makes sense," I ventured.

He paused and went on, "Maggie and I were... well, maybe not on the verge of divorce, but certainly not rooted together. The kids were grown and out of the house, the last one having gone off to college—finally. I say finally because she was a hard one. She was trouble from day one. When Patty was in second grade, we'd reward her for getting fewer than five time-outs at school in a week. Sometimes she'd have more than five in a single day. She was disobedient and defiant and it all came to a head while she was in high school. After all those years of her playing one of us off against the other—especially during her high school years—we were feeling a lot of distance from one another."

"What did you do?" I asked thinking about my youngest who often played the same game with Sara and me.

"We worked on our roots. Not that we called it that, but we—or I should say she—went out of her way to reconnect. Maggie sensed the distance and didn't like it. I was busy with work and didn't pay too much attention, but she couldn't live like that. So she romanced me: flowers in the dining room and kitchen, scented soap in the shower, candles in the bedroom, new recipes, good wine with dinner and," he blushed slightly, "er... lingerie. It took a couple of months, but I started to notice and finally caught on. And once I did, I began inviting her out for dates, weekends, and walks around the neighborhood."

"And it all grew roots?"

"Yes, it did. You see the time together provided spaces in which we could talk. With our kids, we hadn't done too much of that for years. Instead we exchanged information. When you have kids you need to do a lot of that, but once they're gone, a new opportunity opens up. You either take that opportunity and learn to talk—to share about being pears and a grape vines—or you crank at each other and watch a lot of television."

"Or you become a patio guy," I added.

"And that's certainly an option too. What's sad to me is that so many of our friends picked one of those options. The kids went go off and—another cliché—they found they were living with strangers. So rather than getting to know the familiar stranger next to them in bed they found new strangers to get to know."

"You mean they divorced," I added.

"Some did and married their new strangers. Others stayed together, but remained at a distance while getting to know new friends—golf partners, bridge clubs, neighbors, law partners, young mistresses, or whoever. Many—married, divorced, or remarried—just got lonely."

"And bitter?" I added.

"Oh, yes." He went on, "One fellow I knew at my office was sixty-five when the doctor told him he needed triple bypass surgery. He had divorced his wife years earlier, had little contact with his kids, and headed for the hospital and open-heart surgery alone. Can you imagine that? No one to be there when he got out. No one to come home to. No one to take care of him. And how many times does that get repeated in this world?"

He took another sip of wine, savored it, and swallowed. "Do you have any idea how long many people my age sleep? I've known people my age who get ten hours of sleep at night and take a three-hour nap in the middle of the day. It's not because they need the rest. They're lonely even in a home with their husband or wife. There are no roots or maybe I should say there are withered roots that could, with some effort, live again. After all, most people choose a spouse for a reason. What made you want to marry Sara to begin with? Go back to the roots and make them grow. Start now so when you're my age, the roots will be flourishing."

I thought about Sara and how much information we exchange. "I'm not sure where to begin," I said.

"You keep saying that. I'll bet you said it a hundred times about these journals," he answered. "It just took you a while to figure out that there's no right place to start and then you started."

"Yeah, it was like that," I chuckled. "Just start."

"Exactly. It doesn't matter where you start, it only matters *that* you start. You've got years of experience with your wife and you know a great deal more than you think. Draw on that experience and knowledge and just start."

I munched a date and thought for a minute. "Our twenty-fourth anniversary is coming up in a month. I could make reservations to go to an inn we know."

"That's the idea," he said. "What are you doing for number twenty-five."

"Sara wants to go to Tuscany. I guess we could spend part of the weekend discussing next year's trip."

"Ah," he smiled, "then you really do know where to begin." He went on. "The same applies to the rest of your family."

"My kids," I said.

"Your kids, your brothers and sisters, your parents, aunts, uncles, nieces, nephews and cousins. Most people my age and even your age grew up in regular contact with their family. Now everyone's spread across the map and connecting for many people doesn't seem that important. Do you send your first cousins Christmas cards?"

"Uh, no, I don't."

"It's time to start."

"I feel like I have enough problems keeping up with my own kids that I never even think about my cousins—who, of course, all have their own kids."

"Well," he began, "Then let's start where you are, with your own kids. My impression is that you have, in general, a good relationship with them. It's one thing when there's war at home till they leave; it's another when they're transitioning from being your kids to being your friends. That's what the teen years are about after all. They need to step away a bit before they come back and yours are doing that right now."

"But what do I do in the meanwhile?"

"Be a pear, be a grape vine, and be a date palm. You should grow up as much as you can, keep the communication lines open, and share bits and pieces of what you've learned: the good memories that come up as you write in your journal and talk with Sara and the stupid—dare I say, sinful—things you did when they were growing up. Confession and repentance when they're appropriate surprise kids. And hearing you say you screwed up is good for their souls as well as yours."

He paused. "Friends of mine had a son who, after a rocky adolescence, went to college out of state and then got a job out of the country. And, of course, the geographical distance led to relational distance. After the son married a girl they had only met a couple of times they felt very distant. But later the young couple moved nearby and now they stop at mom and dad's for dinner or dessert or just to watch TV. With their daughter living at home and working, they all spend time together as adults. My friends tell me that these are some of the best years of that family's life. Another mother I know meets her three daughters and one daughter-in-law at a spa every year for a long weekend. Those five are spread out across the states, but they take the time to talk, laugh, cry, and pamper themselves. And big family holiday gatherings are, for many, a thing of the past, but a thing of the past that needs to be revived along with family Sunday dinners and all sorts of other rituals that root us in family."

We sat quietly listening to the birds in the garden, sipping wine, and eating cheeses and dates.

"But you know," he said, "you need more than your family. You need friends and community. At least that was my experience and the experience of quite a number of my friends. A whole group of us went 'over the hill' together."

"Do you mean a formal group?"

"Yeah, although 'formal' might imply more organization than we had." He paused, "Here's what happened. A couple of months before I turned fifty, a neighbor named Harvey committed suicide. He calmly left work early one day, went home, drank half a bottle of Scotch, and blew his brains out."

I winced.

"Now, we knew Harvey and his wife fairly well. Maggie and I went to the theater with them more than once and Harvey and I played tennis together with some regularity. In fact, there was a whole group of us who lived in town and had kids about the same ages. So we all knew Harvey and each other from school events, town politics, kids' sports, and what not. His death was a huge shock to my system and I remember sitting there at the funeral looking at that closed box wondering who was next. And it scared the… well, let's just say it scared the *snot* out of me."

"What did you do?" I asked.

"I sat down and wrote a letter," he replied. "I sent it to about thirty men in town who, again, knew each other from community activities. In the letter I told them how I felt: not only the shock, but the utter terror—it was much more than fear by then. I told them that I didn't want to be next and I didn't want any of them to be next. And I suggested a solution: that we band together and support each other."

"And they joined your group?"

"First, it was never meant to be *my* group. I just got it going. Second, only eight joined up. But eight was more than enough and we began meeting together."

"How did they all fit that into their schedules?" I asked, knowing what my schedule and everyone else's looks like. "I know I couldn't add another weekly meeting."

"We talked about that. For some people meeting weekly works, but not with this group. We were like you: too busy for that. Instead we decided to meet two weekends a year. So every six months, we go to a hotel or a beach house or a retreat center."

"You 'go'? Are you still meeting with the original eight?"

"No, five have died and three new men have been added. That makes six."

"No one moved away?"

"Oh, in twenty-five years people have moved quite a bit. That's the advantage of meeting over a weekend. The Californians and one who lives in Las Vegas can still be a part."

"What do you talk about?"

"Life, I guess. We all read the same book before we come and that's the starting point—unless, of course, there's another starting point. We've been through those deaths I mentioned, through two divorces, the death of a spouse, the death of a child, bankruptcy, chemotherapy, open-heart surgery, and just about everything else you can think of."

"So you support each other through the hard times," I said.

"When the wind blows, you've got to have roots to hold you down." He ate a date. "But don't think it's all about weeping and wailing together. We've done more than our share of celebrating too. There have been weddings, new jobs, new homes, kids have stopped using drugs—one guy celebrated fifty years of sobriety. It's been more fun than I can tell you despite the sad events. Deserts where date palms live may be dry and adverse places, but if you spend time there you soon begin to realize that they're full of life and very beautiful. At the risk of sounding trite, the world is just like that: dry and adverse, but beautiful and full of life."

"So, you think I should start a group too?" I asked.

"I think you should be like a date palm and grow deep roots. How you do that is up to you. A group helped me and so I'm passing that on. It may help you. But let me mention two other things.

First, I decided not to move. I'm part of a generation of big company employees who got moved every two years. Once we got here, Maggie and I decided we were sick of moving and decided not to move again. When the company told me to move, I said, no. And much to my surprise, they let me stay. That gave me confidence so that two years later when my number was up again I said, no, again. And to my surprise they fired me." He laughed. "Of course, I wasn't laughing then. I thought I was safe and hadn't done much networking to find something new."

"Did you look long?" I asked.

"About a year. Then I took something that I thought was below me, but it was all I had. As it turned out, I was right. It was below me and boring, but it led to something that was perfect—four years later."

He took another sip. "I'm not saying never move, just that I found that community roots are worth having, community roots and church roots."

I new John went to church and I figured that sooner or later he'd get around to his religion. I really didn't want to hear it, but wanted to be polite.

"You don't go to church, do you?" he asked.

"No," I replied. "I'm a card-carrying, burned-out, non-practicing, ex-Presbyterian."

"Can I encourage you to try it again for the first time? There's that old poem I mentioned that begins, 'Remember your Creator in the days of your youth before the days of trouble come and the years approach when you will say, "I find no pleasure in them."' That's good advice.

"I mentioned that our group of eight is down to six, but it would only be three if we hadn't added some more. And yet we're still down by 25%. Before long it will be 50%, 75%, and then there will only be one left. I have lots of new, young friends—you for instance—but I miss those five old pals who have died. My deep roots were wrapped tightly around them and around Maggie. If the day comes when I'm the only one left, I don't want to be alone. I want to have roots in Someone much bigger than me who will never go away or let me go. I'm convinced that we were designed that way, restless, as another old man once said, until we find our rest in God."

We sat for a few minutes in silence until the clock on the mantle chimed six and I started. "It's already six?" I said.

"That old clock never lies," he replied. "You need to get home to Sara."

"I really do. The afternoon went by too quickly. There's probably more to be said about dates."

"Indeed, there is, the best and sweetest thing."

"Let me call Sara and tell her I'll be a little later than I expected. That is, if it's okay with you."

"I'd be delighted for you to stay," said John.

I knew I'd be out of town quite a bit the next few weeks and I wanted to know the rest of his story about dates. So I called Sara while he walked into the kitchen to replenish the plate of dates and cheese.

DATES AND SWEETNESS

Grow old along with me!
The best is yet to be,
The last of life, for which the first was made.
            —Robert Browning

"The last thing to remember about dates," he said returning from the kitchen, "has to do with age and sweetness. Apple trees—or pear trees for that matter—produce good fruit for only a relatively short number of years. Once they're past their prime, the quality of the fruit deteriorates. A tree that once produced crunchy, sweet apples will, over time, produce nothing but hard bitter fruit.

"I remember years ago when Maggie and I were first married we took a trip to her family's island in Maine. Her great-great-great-great (at least) grandfather homesteaded it in 1804 and it's been in the family ever since. My kids still go up there and I went with them last summer. It's a wonderful place. Of course now it's just a family vacation spot, all wooded over, but that's not how it used to be. They used to farm it. When Maggie's father and her aunts were children, the family went up every summer to work the place. And one of the things they did was plant an apple orchard.

"During my first visit to the island, barely six months after we were married, Maggie saw some fruit on the two old apple trees that were still around. It was August and summer was fading fast up there. She got all excited and decided to show me her skills as a baker by making me an apple pie in the old wood stove."

"Do you mean on top of the stove?"

"No, not at all. It was one of those late 1800's kitchen stoves with an oven. You've probably seen them in movies about that era and never noticed. It looked like a desk with a chimney."

"Oh, of course," I said. "I just never thought of them having an oven."

"Sure," he replied, "How do you think they baked pies for the county fair?"

We laughed and each grabbed another date.

"She had me climb the tree to collect the apples."

"Of course."

"Of course. And I nearly fell out by stepping on a rotten branch that looked for all the world like a sound limb."

"Of course," I said.

"And that should have been a warning. Anyway, I picked the apples and she brought them into the kitchen, peeled them, cored them, sliced them up, and put them in the piecrust with butter, sugar, cinnamon, nutmeg, and raisins. We fed the stove as she worked and the oven was good and hot when she put the pie in."

"By then," I said, "you were mad with anticipation."

"We all were: me and Maggie and her parents and her younger sisters who were on the island with us—actually, knowing her father as I do, I should say we were all on the island with him. Anyway, it was an ancient stove and I'm not sure how hot it ever got, but we dutifully fed it wood and, later rather than sooner, the crust was golden and the pie was ready.

"As the primary object of the baker's affection, once it cooled on the window sill, I got the first taste. It was one of those times when I wished she had shown more deference to her father."

"Oh, no," I said.

"Oh, yes," he replied, "I took one taste of that pie and went rushing outside to spit it out. It was as bitter and vile a thing as I have ever put into my mouth. We never tasted the apples from those trees before baking them. If we had, it would have saved a lot of time and wood. They were apples, but they were apples from an old tree and even hogs wouldn't eat them."

"Okay," I said, "so what's that got to do with dates?"

"Well," he began, "if apple trees were like date trees, that apple pie would have been the sweetest apple pie in history. As apple trees get old, the quality and quantity of fruit diminishes. When date palms get old, their fruit becomes more abundant and sweeter with every passing year. And life for anyone living near the date palm gets sweeter every year. So not only should you be like a date palm because it's rooted deeply in its place, you should be like a date palm because you anticipate, expect, that as you age you'll bear sweeter and sweeter fruit. Anticipation of sweet fruit in old age—that's the second lesson of the date palm.

"You think old age should be sweet?" I asked.

"You weren't listening. I didn't quite say old age is

sweet," he replied. "There's plenty about getting older that's hard to swallow. Maggie's dead. That's still a fact of my life even though it happened years ago. I still roll over at night and wake up wondering where she's gone until I remember exactly where she's gone.

"What I said is that we should anticipate that we'll bear sweeter and sweeter *fruit* in old age and that's an entirely different statement. The desert where the date palm lives is a harsh place. The trees endure scorching sun, high winds, and sandstorms. It's not a sweet life. But the fruit is sweet and gets sweeter as the tree ages. Regardless of your condition as you age, anticipate that you will bear sweet fruit for others."

"But what if…?" I began and then went silent.

"What if what?" John asked.

"I guess I'm still stuck on being a burden and making everyone's life something less than sweet—making it downright miserable."

"That really does bother you." He paused, "Let me answer it this way. My daddy had a workbench in our basement and on that workbench was a cigar box about a quarter filled with ball bearings. I loved that box full of little metal balls. It made a wonderful noise when you shook it and I used to try to build with the ball bearings. I even made a few very short pyramids, but they always fell down.

"My impression is that most people – including you – think of human beings as ball bearings. We're individuals, hard and strong. We interact with each other the way ball bearings do in a cigar box by running into each other and occasionally forming a bit of a pyramid, but rolling apart again. And everything goes along fine until one of the ball bearings has needs he can't take care of on his own. Suddenly he's a burden to the others and they're all too busy being hard individuals to care for the one in need."

"I admit that I see it that way. Isn't that the way it is?" I asked.

"Well," he replied, "that may be how it is, but it's not the way it should be. Human beings, as I've said, aren't independent and self-sufficient. You and I are never like ball bearings simply colliding with others and never being a burden. We always need others, we always make demands of others, and we're always something of a burden. We're not machines; we're people and, as the song goes, 'People who need people are the luckiest people in the world.'"

"I know what you said about the need for a trellis, but I'm not sure that or your ball bearing story helps," I replied.

"How about this," he began again. "I've never cared for someone who's sick for years and years the way some folks do, but I cared for Maggie for six months as she died of cancer. Now she was always the one caring for others and suddenly she had to lie there and have others care for her. She didn't like it one bit. She was embarrassed, ashamed, and, in the final analysis, angry as all get out. I helped her in and out of bed, dressed her, washed her, fed her, and got her whatever she needed. She struggled with it before she finally acquiesced, but I didn't struggle at all. There was something ennobling about caring for someone as fine and good as Maggie. She felt as though she was a burden—even talked about wanting to overdose on morphine to get away from that feeling—but she was never a burden to me. Oh, some days maybe, but overall…, well, there really is such a thing as a labor of love. And I think labors of love are easier to do than they are to receive. At least that's my experience. Even in her need, even when it wasn't sweet

Pears, Grapes, and Dates

to her, Maggie's life was sweet to me."

For a while neither of us said anything. Finally I asked, "How do I bear sweet fruit?"

"Well, partly," he began, "you bear sweet fruit by being a pear, a grape vine, and a date palm: <u>ripening from the inside out, pruning away what doesn't belong, and rooting yourself</u>. But that's not enough. You have to want to and expect to bear sweet fruit."

He took another swallow of wine, "Look, most people as they age think to themselves, 'I've worked hard all my life. I've cleared the land, plowed, planted, tended, and now it's time to reap my reward. The fruit of my labor belongs to me.' And so they gather everything up for themselves into huge barns so they can live out their days in comfort, and—only too often—self-indulgence. Now, not everybody does that and we all do it a little, but that's the trend I see.

"I had an eighty-some year old gentleman wallpaper one of my bathrooms years ago when we lived in years ago Florida. He was from up north somewhere and had been in the wallpapering business since he was a teenager. Finally he sold the business, retired, and moved to a retirement community. So why, I asked him, was he out wallpapering again? Do you know what he said?"

"No," I answered.

"He told me that soon after he and his wife moved down, they were invited to a neighbor's house for a dinner party. Dinner, he said, plus lots of booze. The evening dragged on and he kept wondering when everyone was going to go home. Finally they all left at about 2 in the morning. As they walked home from the party with another couple, the fellow asked him, 'Do you want to come to our house for a nightcap?' 'A nightcap?' he asked in shock. 'Sure,' said his neighbor, 'none of us have anything to do tomorrow, so why not?'

"Within a week he had business cards, an old, faded, blue van, and a pile of wallpapering tools. He found something to do in the morning. Better yet, he found a way to be fruitful."

"Did he do a good job?" I asked.

"A good job? Friend, he had more than sixty years of wallpapering experience under his belt. He did a stunning job with what turned out to be really cheap wallpaper that I'd bought. He was also a happy man as he shared the sweet fruit of his life with our family by making our bathroom look lovely.

"You see, we work hard throughout our lives clearing the land, plowing, planting, and tending. Now that it's time to reap, the goal is to allow others to enjoy the sweet harvest. Filling up big barns at my age—really at any age—is foolish, an exercise in futility."

"But didn't you work and save for a comfortable retirement? Shouldn't everyone? It seems to me that it's only prudent."

"Well," he said scratching his cheek, "maybe I'm overstating. Here's what I'm getting at: It's not what you have; it's how you handle it and what you do with it. As we harvest the fruit and stuff it into bigger and bigger barns, we need to remember that we're mortal. You may die tonight and—more likely than that—*I* may die tonight. Then what happens to all my hard work, all I've worked for and held onto?"

He stretched a bit and poured us both the last drops from the bottle of wine.

"An old saying says that it may go to someone who will use it wisely or it may go to a fool who will squander it all. And I'm not saying we should spend or give away our children's inheritance. I don't think that's right. But neither do I think we should spend our old age in self-indulgent behavior.

"I went on a cruise with my kids and their families a year or so ago. I met some wonderful people my own age." He laughed, "Had my first date in more than half a century. Lovely woman. I still correspond with a little group—including the lady. But I watched others my age who, it seemed, were only interested in their next meal. One woman named Pearl summed it up. I'll never forget what she said: 'What's mine is mine to spend on my self and that's exactly what I'm going to do.' That approach is a guaranteed way to live a lonely old age because enough is never enough if all you do is think about yourself.

"Compare that with a friend of mine who, in her seventies, visits prisoners, works with inner-city kids, raises money for good causes, and runs her own business. Or a woman who even though she was poor, infirmed, and lived in a rundown retirement home, was filled with joy in her old age writing to and praying for dozens of prisoners every week. Or another friend who is also in his seventies and works with high school kids at her church and serves as a hospice volunteer."

"But isn't that a habit of thinking that goes back to early life?"

"Oh certainly," he agreed. "That's why we've talked about pears, grapes and dates—ripening from the inside out, pruning away bitterness, and being rooted. As we age we become more and more who we already are. If we're self-centered or bitter or mean at age thirty, we'll be more self-centered, bitter, and mean by age fifty."

"And at age seventy?" I asked.

"At age seventy we'll be worse. Oh, and we'll also be lonely and miserable to top it off. But if we're learning gratitude, pruning away bitterness, and are increasingly rooted in the lives of others, we'll be increasingly joyful people."

"That's rather motivating," I said.

"It should be," he replied. "You're at a crucial point. Too many people my age checked out long ago. Either they became increasingly self-centered and self-indulgent or they came to believe that they were 'old and in the way' so they gave up. Don't do either. You're a date palm. Expect that you'll bear sweeter and sweeter fruit every year. And don't forget, it's fruit for others, not for you, which means you need to consider how you can sweeten the lives of those around you. If I've learned anything in my dotage (as it were)," his eyes twinkled, "it's that when I'm giving to others, being fruitful for them, their lives are sweeter and—as a bonus—mine becomes sweeter as well."

"But," I said, "at the risk of being a cynic, don't others take advantage? The philosopher Jean Paul Sarte said, 'Hell is other people,' and while that may not always be the case…"

"Jean Paul Sarte was an old crank," he interrupted. "While it's true that some people are, in fact, Hell, most people aren't. Most people are just trying to get by and if you and I can help them, why wouldn't we? If we can be a source of refreshing sweetness, isn't that our business as fellow humans? And the older we get, the more time we have to be sweet and the more we have to offer. I've walked the stretch of the road you're walking today. I think I have something to offer you to make your way easier and sweeter. And you keep coming back to listen so I assume I must be correct."

"Absolutely, John. I can't tell you how helpful you've been. My journals are filling up, I've lost some weight, and I'm taking my wife out on a date tomorrow night."

"And, I hope, you've just begun. Don't believe that it's only the young who count. We old codgers have plenty to offer—in fact, because we've seen it all, we have *more* to offer. The pity is that most of us don't know it or don't value it and so we settle for far less."

The phone rang and John got up to answer it. "Yes, your long lost spouse is still in my living room," he said. There was a pause. "Why I'd love to make sure he gets home soon and stay for dinner. Ah-huh. Okay, I'll tell him. Bye-bye, see you in about ten minutes, Sara. Okay."

"You're wanted at home and we're all having oven seared salmon with loganberry sauce for dinner. Let me walk down to my wine cellar and then I'll make sure you're home on time." He laughed and disappeared down the cellar stairs.

EPILOGUE

Age is strictly a case of mind over matter. If you don't mind, it doesn't matter.
—Jack Benny

One Saturday morning about two months later, the phone rang.

"Jeff?" the voice on the other end said.

"Yes."

"This is Patty, John Freeman's daughter. It's about dad," she said.

My stomach dropped. "Is he in the hospital?" I replied thinking that it must be some health problem.

"No," she answered. "Haven't you heard? He's getting married. We have to do something."

There was no helping myself. Patty was clearly upset and I made matters worse. All I could do was laugh for joy.

I called John and left a message on his machine congratulating him and wondering if Sara and I could drop by with a bottle of champagne. Before he could return the call, the mail arrived. It included an invitation.

Mr. & Mrs. Richard Locke

(if they were still living would be amazed to)

Invite You To Attend

The Wedding of Their Daughter

Barbara Jean Locke Rostov

To

John William Freeman

On September 25

10:30 O'clock AM

First Church of Providence

Reception to Follow at the Church

RSVP

The phone rang. "Jeff? This is John. Can the two of

you come over and meet my bride."

Sara and I headed to John's and heard the whole story. That date on the cruise that he had mentioned to me led to letters, phone calls, visits, and romance. "We can't quite believe it ourselves," said John. "But it's wonderful, just wonderful."

The wedding was beyond all I expected. I've been to many weddings at that church. The thousand-seat sanctuary usually looks very empty. This wedding was different. The pews were packed with a standing room only crowd spilling out of the doors in back.

The ages ranged from teenagers to octogenarians—friends with all kinds of connections to John and Barbara. I spoke with a group of six young men and women who knew John from the local supermarket where he shopped. A ragged old man who lived in the park came and stood in the very back. John used to talk to him and sometimes brought him sandwiches, he said. And he had never been invited to anything for years. A delegation came from the police department and a dozen fifth-graders sat with their parents near the front—John's Sunday school class. All these people—plus most of his church—had come to celebrate John and Barbara's wedding and, very clearly, to celebrate and sing praises to God for the goodness of a ripe, well-pruned, rooted, and sweet life.

The reception that followed was a simple one, hors d'oeuvres, lemonade, and cake. The couple greeted their guests and then, at 1:30 Sara and I drove them to the airport to fly to Miami and a honeymoon cruise. "Now that ships have double beds," said John, "they make great places for honeymoons."

That evening I sat down to reflect on the day, the service, and my friendship with John. This is what I wrote:

As medical science progresses, we're all living longer and longer and yet there is greater and greater distance between people. It's easy to live a long life. The goal is to live a full life, the kind of life John has. He's full of years and full of friends, sweetening the lives of those around him. Now it's my turn. I'll do what I can to ripen from the inside out like a pear, to prune away the excess like a grape vine, bear others' burdens while I let them bear mine, and root myself like a date palm. Then may God grant me the fruitfulness of old age that I see in my friend John and make my life a sweet blessing to everyone I meet.

ABOUT THE AUTHOR

Dr. James Tonkowich is a freelance writer, speaker, and commentator on spirituality, religion, and public life. He is the author of *The Liberty Threat: The Attack on Religious Freedom in America Today* from St. Benedict Press and has contributed to a wide variety of opinion websites and publications. Jim also serves as Special Advisor to the President for Strategic Initiatives at Wyoming Catholic College. Jim and Dottie have been blissfully married for nearly forty years. They have one son, a wonderful daughter-in-law, and two fantastic grandchildren. Jim's other work can be found at www.JimTonkowich.com.

Made in the USA
Middletown, DE
15 March 2015